CKD STAGE 5 COOKBOOK FOR BEGINNERS

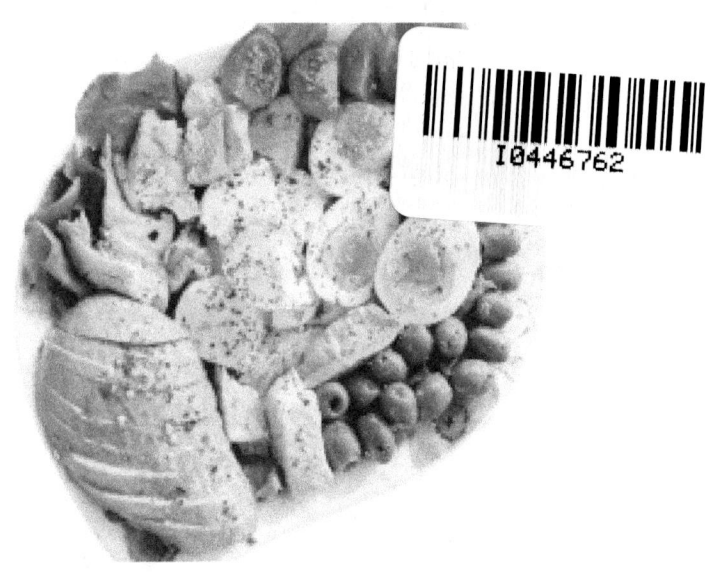

The Ultimate Guide With Quick and Easy Low Sodium and Potassium Recipes to Manage And Reverse Chronic Renal Disease Stage 5

THERESA EATON

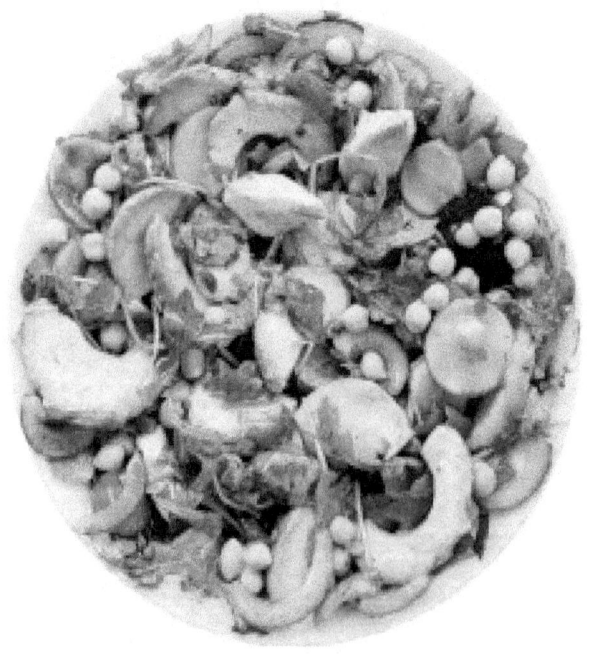

Table of Contents

INTRODUCTION

Understanding your body's demands is critical in the field of health and well-being. This understanding is especially important for people who are traversing the difficult road of Chronic Kidney Disease (CKD) Stage 5. End-stage renal Disease (ESRD), also known as CKD Stage 5, affects millions of individuals worldwide, affecting the way their kidneys handle waste and fluid.

CKD Stage 5 occurs when the kidneys have lost nearly all of their function. Diabetes, hypertension, autoimmune illnesses, and other conditions can all contribute to this syndrome. Its symptoms may be minor at first, but they deteriorate over time, leaving people weary, bloated, anaemic, and with a disrupted mineral and bone metabolism.

Dietary management becomes a keystone in the search for greater health and a higher quality of life at this critical period. The foods we eat have an indisputable impact on CKD management and symptom relief. This is where the book comes in.

The Importance of A Kidney-Friendly Diet

It's not just about the nutrients in a kidney-friendly diet; it's about empowerment, healing, and embracing the potential of a better future. It is all about making educated decisions that can not only decrease the course of CKD but also enhance the quality of life.

Our Book's Goal

This book, "CKD Stage 5 Cookbook for Beginners," will be your constant companion on the path to a better, happier life with CKD Stage 5. Our goal is simple yet profound: to give practical, delicious recipes and assistance customized exclusively for novices who are just starting in the world of kidney-friendly eating.

If you've recently been diagnosed with CKD Stage 5 or are assisting a loved one on their health journey, this book will provide you with hope, inspiration, and gastronomic joy. We will delve into the science of kidney health, walk you through the process of creating a kidney-friendly kitchen, and provide you with delectable dishes that demonstrate that eating properly with CKD Stage 5 can be a tasty experience.

Welcome to a new chapter in your life, one in which your food choices will be your most powerful friends in the fight against CKD. Let's go on this adventure together, where every mouthful leads to a better, happier you.

CHAPTER 1

Did you know that chronic kidney disease (CKD) affects more than 700 million individuals worldwide? It's a figure that illustrates the disease's global impact. You are not alone if you or a loved one have been diagnosed with CKD Stage 5. Understanding CKD Stage 5 and its complexities is the first step toward better renal health and a higher quality of life.

What is CKD Stage 5?

CKD Stage 5, also known as End-Stage Renal Disease (ESRD), is the most severe and advanced stage of chronic kidney disease. At this point, the kidneys have lost practically all of their function, leaving persons highly dependent on dialysis or a kidney transplant to survive. Understanding the underlying causes, symptoms, and potential consequences of CKD Stage 5 is critical for properly managing this illness.

Causes, Symptoms, and Complications of CKD Stage 5

Long-term hypertension, uncontrolled diabetes, autoimmune illnesses, and hereditary factors can all contribute to CKD Stage 5.

Understanding the origin of your CKD is critical since it might affect your therapy and dietary control.

The symptoms of CKD Stage 5 might be mild in the early stages, but they tend to worsen over time. Common symptoms include fatigue, oedema, difficulty sleeping, changes in urine, and anaemia.

Furthermore, CKD Stage 5 comes with a slew of possible problems. These can include issues with bone health, heart disease, and fluid excess. Managing these issues necessitates a multifaceted strategy, which frequently includes dietary changes.

Dietary Planning in Stage 5 CKD

The kidneys serve an important role in maintaining the body's internal environment by regulating electrolytes, eliminating waste products, and controlling blood pressure. When the kidneys are severely injured, the functions are impaired, making it vital to control what you eat. A well-planned, kidney-friendly diet can help delay the course of CKD, control symptoms, and improve overall health.

It is strongly advised to engage closely with a registered dietitian specializing in renal health to negotiate the complexities of dietary management in CKD Stage 5. These specialists have the expertise and experience to build individualized nutritional regimens that are tailored to your unique needs and tastes.

Overview of Dietary Restrictions: Potassium, Phosphorus, and Sodium

One of the fundamental goals of a kidney-friendly diet is to control important nutrients such as potassium, phosphorus, and salt. When the kidneys are unable to eliminate these minerals adequately, they might build up in the circulation. We'll go into more detail about these constraints in upcoming chapters, but it's critical to appreciate their significance and how they affect your everyday life.

In the next chapters, we'll look at the practical aspects of establishing a kidney-friendly diet, from setting up your kidney-friendly kitchen to making tasty meals that adhere to your dietary requirements. You are not alone on this path, and together we will take the initial steps toward a better, more vibrant life with CKD Stage 5.

CHAPTER 2

Setting Up Your Kidney-Friendly Kitchen

Did you know that a well-equipped kitchen might be your secret weapon in the fight against CKD Stage 5? To produce delectable, kidney-friendly dishes, a seasoned cook, like a warrior, needs the right tools. In this chapter, we'll go over the important elements of your culinary armoury and lay the groundwork for your culinary path to greater kidney health.

Essential Kitchen Utensils and Tools

Every cook, regardless of expertise, relies on a set of vital equipment. In your case, making a kidney-friendly kitchen begins with:

1. **Nonstick Cookware:** Choose nonstick pans and pots to decrease the need for extra oil, making it easier to make meals with less additional fat.

2. **Food scale:** Precision is essential for portion management and exact measuring of components. A food scale is your go-to for keeping track of portion amounts.

3. **Slow Cooker:** A slow cooker is a useful equipment for creating kidney-friendly stews, soups, and casseroles since it allows for extended, slow cooking without the use of excessive salt.

4. **Renal Diet Cookbook Stand:** Invest in a stand that supports your cookbook or recipe card as you cook, leaving your hands free and your kitchen tidy.

Reading Food Labels for Nutritional Data

The act of reading food labels is a skill set that will enable you to make informed purchasing and eating decisions. Look out for:

- **Sodium content:** High sodium levels might contribute to fluid retention and elevated blood pressure. Look for low-sodium or no-salt-added alternatives.

- **Potassium and Phosphorus:** Monitor the potassium and phosphorus content, as these minerals are frequently restricted in a CKD-friendly diet.

- **Hidden Phosphorus:** Be wary of chemicals such as phosphoric acid, which can surreptitiously boost your phosphorus consumption.

Tips for Safe Food Preparation and Storage

1. **Washing Instructions:** Wash fruits and vegetables thoroughly to limit the chance of eating hazardous germs and pollutants.

2. **Cutting Boards and Utensils:** To avoid cross-contamination, use separate cutting boards and utensils for raw meat and fresh veggies.

3. **Safe Food Temperatures:** Cook food at safe temperatures, especially when working with meats, to kill any hazardous germs.

4. **Food Storage:** To ensure freshness and safety, store perishable goods in the refrigerator or freezer as soon as possible.

Meal Planning for CKD Stage 5

Meal planning is essential for CKD Stage 5 nutritional treatment. You can ensure that you always have kidney-friendly foods on hand by prepping meals ahead of time. This lessens the temptation to go for unhealthy snacks or order fast food when you're pressed for time.

In the next chapters, we'll get into the practicalities of making delicious, kidney-friendly breakfasts, lunches, and dinners, as well as sensible snacking and gratifying sweet delights. Your kidney-friendly kitchen is where it all begins, and with the correct equipment and knowledge, you'll be well on your way to culinary success in managing CKD Stage 5.

CHAPTER 3

Did you know that starting your day with a kidney-friendly breakfast can improve your overall health? Breakfast is generally referred to be the most essential meal of the day, and with good reason. In this chapter, we'll discuss the importance of a substantial, kidney-friendly breakfast and give you a range of tasty and healthy meals to get your day started.

The Importance of a Hearty Breakfast

A well-balanced breakfast is like a gentle wake-up call for your body, announcing the start of a new day and offering the energy you need to face it with excitement. When you have CKD Stage 5, a kidney-friendly breakfast is critical for maintaining stable blood sugar levels and keeping your energy levels up throughout the day.

Kidney-friendly Breakfast Basics

Consider the following concepts for a kidney-friendly breakfast:

1. **Protein-Packed Options:** Incorporate high-quality, low-phosphorus proteins such as egg whites, tofu, and lean cuts of meat.

2. **Low-Potassium Fruits:** While fresh fruits are delicious, choose low-potassium selections such as berries, apples, and pears.

3. **Reduced Sodium:** Excess sodium in your breakfast might influence blood pressure and fluid balance.

Recipes

Easy Turkey Breakfast Burrito

Preparation Time: 15 minutes

Servings: 2

Ingredients:
- 4 large egg whites
- 2 small whole-grain tortillas
- 4 ounces ground turkey, cooked and seasoned
- 1/4 cup diced bell peppers
- 1/4 cup diced onions
- Salt and pepper to taste
- 1/4 cup low-sodium salsa

Preparation:

1. Sauté the chopped bell peppers and onions in a nonstick pan until soft.

2. Add the cooked ground turkey to the pan and thoroughly warm it.

3. Whisk the egg whites and scramble them in the skillet until done.

4. Adjust the seasoning using salt and pepper to taste.

5. Divide the mixture among the tortillas, top with salsa, and wrap into burritos.

Nutritional Information (per serving):

Calories: Approximately 230 Protein: 20g Carbohydrates: 21g

Fiber: 3g Fat: 7g Potassium: 320mg Phosphorus: 220mg Sodium: 370mg

Chocolate Pancakes with Moon Pie Stuffing

Preparation Time: 30 minutes

Servings: 2

Ingredients:

- 1/2 cup whole-grain pancake mix (low-phosphorus)

- 1/2 cup unsweetened almond milk

- 2 tablespoons unsweetened cocoa powder

- 1 tablespoon honey
- 1/2 cup low-phosphorus marshmallow fluff
- 1/4 cup crushed graham crackers (low-phosphorus)

Preparation:
- Make the pancake mix following the package directions, then add the chocolate powder.
- Prepare the chocolate pancakes by cooking them.
- Distribute marshmallow fluff on one pancake, then sprinkle with broken graham crackers before topping with another.
- Serve and enjoy.

Nutritional Information (per serving):

Calories: Approximately 330 Protein: 5g Carbohydrates: 65g

Fiber: 4g Fat: 8g Potassium: 90mg Phosphorus: 85mg Sodium: 190mg

Blueberry Muffins

Preparation Time: 30 minutes

Servings: 6

Ingredients:

- 1 cup low-phosphorus baking mix
- 1/4 cup unsweetened applesauce
- 1/4 cup unsweetened almond milk
- 1/2 cup fresh blueberries
- 1/4 cup honey
- 1/2 teaspoon vanilla extract

Preparation:

1. Prepare the muffin tray by lining it with paper liners and setting up the oven to 350°F (175°C).
2. Put together the baking mix, applesauce, almond milk, honey, and vanilla extract in a large mixing dish.
3. Fold in the blueberries carefully.
4. Fill the muffin cups halfway with the batter.
5. Bake for about twenty to twenty-five till a toothpick inserted into the middle comes out clean.
6. Serve and enjoy.

Nutritional Information (per serving):

Calories: Approximately 130 Protein: 2g Carbohydrates: 28g

Fiber: 2g Fat: 1g Potassium: 90mg Phosphorus: 50mg Sodium: 140mg

Spicy Tofu Scrambler

Preparation Time: 20 minutes

Servings: 2

Ingredients:

- 1/2 block of extra-firm tofu, crumbled
- 1/4 cup diced bell peppers
- 1/4 cup diced onions
- 1/2 teaspoon turmeric (for colour)
- 1/2 teaspoon chilli powder
- Salt and pepper to taste
- 1 tablespoon olive oil
- 2 tablespoons chopped fresh cilantro

Preparation:

1. Using a skillet over a moderate amount of heat, heat the olive oil.
2. Add and cook the bell peppers and onions till they are soft.

3. Toss in the crushed tofu, turmeric, chilli powder, salt, and pepper. Cook till heated thoroughly.

4. Add a garnish of fresh cilantro and serve.

Nutritional Information (per serving):

Calories: Approximately 170 Protein: 9g Carbohydrates: 7g

Fiber: 1g Fat: 11g Potassium: 215mg Phosphorus: 95mg Sodium: 120mg

Strawberry Fruit Salad

Preparation Time: 10 minutes

Servings: 2

Ingredients:

- 1 cup fresh strawberries, sliced
- 1/2 cup fresh pineapple, diced
- 1/4 cup fresh blueberries
- 1 tablespoon honey (optional)
- Fresh mint leaves for garnish

Preparation:

1. In a mixing dish, combine strawberries, pineapple, and blueberries.

2. If you wish, sprinkle with honey.

3. Top with fresh mint leaves.
4. Serve and enjoy.

Nutritional Information (per serving):

Calories: Approximately 80 Protein: 1g Carbohydrates: 20g
Fiber: 3g Fat: 0g Potassium: 190mg Phosphorus: 20mg Sodium:
0mg

Cranberry Pancakes

Preparation Time: 20 minutes

Servings: 2

Ingredients:

- 1/2 cup low-phosphorus pancake mix
- 1/2 cup unsweetened cranberry juice
- 1/4 cup fresh cranberries
- 1 tablespoon honey (optional)

Preparation:

1. In a mixing dish, combine the pancake mix and cranberry juice.
2. Mix with the fresh cranberries.
3. Cook the pancakes following the package instructions.
4. If you like, sprinkle with honey.

5. Serve and enjoy the cranberry pancakes.

Nutritional Information (per serving):

Calories: Approximately 180 Protein: 3g Carbohydrates: 40g
Fiber: 2g Fat: 1g Potassium: 70mg Phosphorus: 65mg Sodium:
210mg

High Protein Breakfast Tacos

Preparation Time: 15 minutes
Servings: 2

Ingredients:

- 2 whole-grain soft taco shells
- 4 large egg whites
- A half-cup amount of black beans (canned, drained, and rinsed)
- 1/4 cup diced tomatoes
- 2 tablespoons low-fat shredded cheese
- Fresh cilantro for garnish
- Salsa for serving

Preparation:

1. Set aside the egg whites after scrambling them until they are done.

2. Warm the black beans using the microwave or on the stovetop.

3. Split the taco shells with the egg whites, black beans, and chopped tomatoes.

4. Garnish with fresh cilantro and shredded cheese.

5. Serve alongside the salsa on the side.

Nutritional Information (per serving):

Calories: Approximately 280 Protein: 22g Carbohydrates: 31g
Fiber: 7g Fat: 7g Potassium: 370mg Phosphorus: 185mg Sodium:
310mg

Cinnamon Roll Overnight Oats

Preparation Time: 5 minutes (plus overnight soaking)
Servings: 2

Ingredients:

- 1 cup old-fashioned oats
- 1 cup unsweetened almond milk
- 1/2 teaspoon ground cinnamon
- 1/2 teaspoon vanilla extract

- 1 tablespoon honey (optional)
- Chopped pecans for topping (optional)

Preparation:

1. Bring together the oats, almond milk, cinnamon, and vanilla essence in a jar or container.
2. If you want, sweeten it with honey.
3. Place it in the fridge overnight, covered.
4. In the morning, mix thoroughly and top with chopped pecans if desired.

Nutritional Information (per serving):

Calories: Approximately 190 Protein: 5g Carbohydrates: 33g
Fiber: 5g Fat: 4g Potassium: 130mg Phosphorus: 85mg Sodium: 100mg

Vegan Fruit Smoothie

Preparation Time: 10 minutes

Servings: 2

Ingredients:

- 1 cup unsweetened almond milk
- A single cup of fresh blueberries, strawberries and raspberries
- 1/2 banana
- 1/2 cup fresh spinach leaves
- 1 tablespoon honey (optional)
- Ice cubes

Preparation:

1. Use a blender to blend the almond milk, mixed berries, banana, spinach, and ice cubes till smooth.
2. If you want, top and sweeten with honey.
3. Serve and enjoy.

Nutritional Information (per serving):

Calories: Approximately 110 Protein: 2g Carbohydrates: 25g

Fiber: 5g Fat: 2g Potassium: 270mg Phosphorus: 60mg Sodium: 160mg

Fig and Ricotta Toast

Preparation Time: 10 minutes

Servings: 2

Ingredients:

- 2 slices whole-grain bread
- 1/4 cup low-fat ricotta cheese
- 4 fresh figs, sliced
- 1 teaspoon honey (optional)
- Fresh mint leaves for garnish

Preparation:

1. Toast the whole wheat bread till it becomes crispy.
2. On every single piece, spread ricotta cheese.
3. Garnish with fresh fig slices.
4. If you want, spread with honey and top with fresh mint leaves.
5. Serve and enjoy your meal.

Nutritional Information (per serving):

Calories: Approximately 190 Protein: 6g Carbohydrates: 33g

Fiber: 5g Fat: 4g Potassium: 350mg Phosphorus: 120mg Sodium: 200mg

CHAPTER 4

Lunch Recipes

Lunch is a significant time in your day. It's the moment when you replenish your energy and refuel your body, creating the framework for an active, productive afternoon. Crafting balanced and kidney-friendly meals is a key step toward greater health and well-being for persons with CKD Stage 5. This chapter will discuss the significance of these midday meals and give you a variety of scrumptious dishes to keep you motivated.

Significance of Balanced Lunches

Balanced meals are like the gasoline that keeps your engine operating smoothly throughout the day. They provide the necessary nutrients your body requires, and when tailored to your CKD Stage 5 requirements, they are an important component of your overall well-being.

Fundamentals of A Kidney-Friendly Lunch

1. **Protein Variety:** Include a range of high-quality, low-phosphorus proteins, such as tofu, skinless poultry, and beans, to offer energy and help in tissue regeneration.

2. **Fiber and vegetables:** Fiber-rich veggies such as broccoli, zucchini, and cauliflower can help control digestion while also providing vitamins and minerals.

3. **Low-Sodium Seasonings:** Use herbs, spices, and low-sodium seasonings to enhance taste without adding too much salt.

Recipes:

Crunchy Quinoa Salad

Preparation Time: 30 minutes

Servings: 4

Ingredients:

- 1 cup quinoa, cooked and cooled
- 1 cup mixed bell peppers, diced
- 1 cup cucumber, diced
- 1/4 cup red onion, finely chopped
- 1/4 cup fresh parsley, chopped
- 1/4 cup lemon juice
- 2 tablespoons olive oil
- Salt and pepper to taste

Preparation:

1. Combine and mix quinoa, bell peppers, cucumber, red onion, and fresh parsley in a large mixing basin.
2. In a separate bowl, whisk all together the lemon juice, olive oil, salt, and pepper.
3. Transfer the dressing to the quinoa salad and toss with the dressing to coat.
4. Serve and enjoy.

Nutritional Information (per serving):

Calories: Approximately 220 Protein: 6g Carbohydrates: 30g Fiber: 4g Fat: 9g Potassium: 300mg Phosphorus: 100mg Sodium: 70mg

Cucumber Cups Stuffed with Buffalo Chicken Salad

Preparation Time: 20 minutes

Servings: 4

Ingredients:

- 2 cups cooked chicken breast, diced
- 1/4 cup low-fat Greek yogurt
- 2 tablespoons hot sauce (low-sodium)
- 1/4 cup celery, finely chopped

- 1/4 cup carrot, finely chopped
- 2 cucumbers, sliced into cups

Preparation:

1. Bring together the chopped chicken, low-fat Greek yoghurt, spicy sauce, celery, and carrot in a mixing dish.
2. To make cups, scoop off the seeds from the cucumber slices.
3. Stuff the cucumber cups with the buffalo chicken salad.
4. Serve and enjoy.

Nutritional Information (per serving):

Calories: Approximately 160 Protein: 25g Carbohydrates: 3g

Fiber: 1g Fat: 5g Potassium: 200mg Phosphorus: 160mg Sodium: 220mg

Herb-Roasted Chicken Breasts

Preparation Time: 35 minutes

Servings: 2

Ingredients:

- 2 boneless, skinless chicken breasts
- 1 tablespoon olive oil
- 1 teaspoon dried rosemary

- 1 teaspoon dried thyme
- 1 teaspoon dried oregano
- Salt and pepper to taste

Preparation:
1. Set the oven temperature to 375°F (190°C).
2. Season the chicken breasts with dried rosemary, thyme, oregano, salt, and pepper after rubbing them with olive oil.
3. Roast the chicken for twenty-five to thirty up to the point that the internal temperature gets to 165°F (74°C).
4. Bring it out of the oven. Serve and enjoy.

Nutritional Information (per serving):
Calories: Approximately 220 Protein: 40g Carbohydrates: 1g
Fibre: 0g Fat: 6g Potassium: 350mg Phosphorus: 260mg Sodium:
100mg

Lemon Orzo Spring Salad

Preparation Time: 25 minutes

Servings: 4

Ingredients:

- 1 cup orzo pasta (low-phosphorus)
- Zest and juice of 1 lemon
- 1/4 cup extra virgin olive oil
- 1 cup cherry tomatoes, halved
- 1/4 cup fresh basil, chopped
- Salt and pepper to taste

Preparation:

1. Orzo pasta should be cooked according to package guidance, then rinse and allow to cool down.
2. Combine the lemon zest, juice, and extra virgin olive oil in a large mixing basin.
3. The cooked and chilled orzo, cherry tomatoes, and fresh basil should be added now. Toss everything together.
4. Adjust the seasoning using salt and pepper to taste.
5. Serve and enjoy it.

Nutritional Information (per serving):

Calories: Approximately 220 Protein: 4g Carbohydrates: 30g
Fiber: 2g Fat: 9g Potassium: 110mg Phosphorus: 60mg Sodium:
15mg

Mexican Pasta Salad with Creamy Avocado Dressing

Preparation Time: 30 minutes

Servings: 4

Ingredients:

- 2 cups cooked pasta (low-phosphorus)
- 1 cup black beans, drained and rinsed
- 1 cup corn kernels (fresh or frozen)
- 1 cup cherry tomatoes, halved
- 1/4 cup red onion, finely chopped
- 2 ripe avocados, peeled and diced
- 1/4 cup low-fat Greek yogurt
- 2 tablespoons lime juice
- 1 teaspoon chilli powder (low-sodium)
- Salt and pepper to taste

Preparation:

1. Cook the pasta as directed on the package, then strain and allow to cool down.
2. Combine the pasta, black beans, corn, cherry tomatoes, and red onion in a large mixing basin.
3. Mash one avocado in a different dish and blend with low-fat Greek yoghurt, lime juice, chilli powder, salt, and pepper.
4. Toss the pasta salad using the creamy avocado dressing and serve with chopped avocados on top.

Nutritional Information (per serving):

Calories: Approximately 300 Protein: 8g   Carbohydrates: 45g Fiber: 9g Fat: 12g Potassium: 560mg Phosphorus: 150mg Sodium: 30mg

Crispy Cod Sandwich

Preparation Time: 25 minutes

Servings: 2

Ingredients:

- 2 pieces of cod fillet
- 2 whole-grain buns
- 1/4 cup whole-grain breadcrumbs
- 1/4 cup cornmeal
- 1/4 cup low-fat tartar sauce
- Lettuce and tomato slices for garnish

Preparation:

1. Using a small mixing container, bring together the whole-grain breadcrumbs and cornmeal.
2. Using a fork, coat the fish fillets with the breadcrumb mixture.
3. Cook the cod fillets in a nonstick pan on a medium flame until crunchy and done through.
4. Serve the crispy cod fillets on whole-grain buns with lettuce and tomato slices, and low-fat tartar sauce on the side.

Nutritional Information (per serving):

Calories: Approximately 300 Protein: 30g Carbohydrates: 35g Fiber: 5g Fat: 6g Potassium: 450mg Phosphorus: 250mg Sodium: 350mg

Mediterranean Tuna-Spinach Salad

Preparation Time: 20 minutes

Servings: 2

Ingredients:

- 2 cans of low-sodium tuna, drained
- 2 cups fresh spinach leaves
- 1/4 cup Kalamata olives, pitted and sliced
- 1/4 cup red onion, finely chopped
- 1/4 cup feta cheese, crumbled
- 2 tablespoons extra virgin olive oil
- 1 tablespoon balsamic vinegar
- Salt and pepper to taste

Preparation:

1. Combine drained tuna, fresh spinach leaves, Kalamata olives, red onion, and crumbled feta cheese in a large mixing basin.

2. Whisk together the extra virgin olive oil, balsamic vinegar, salt, and pepper using a different bowl.

3. Toss the salad with the dressing to mix it.

4. Serve and enjoy.

Nutritional Information (per serving):
Calories: Approximately 310 Protein: 28gCarbohydrates: 6g

Fiber: 2g Fat: 20g Potassium: 570mg Phosphorus: 250mg Sodium: 320mg

Salmon Pita Sandwich

Preparation Time: 25 minutes

Servings: 2

Ingredients:
- 2 whole-grain pita bread pockets
- 2 grilled salmon fillets
- 1/4 cup low-fat tzatziki sauce
- A single cup of a variety of greens like spinach, arugula, or lettuce
- 1/4 cup cucumber, thinly sliced
- 1/4 cup tomato, diced
- 1/4 cup red onion, thinly sliced

Preparation:

1. Each pita bread pocket should be cut in half to create two pockets.
2. Spread the low-fat tzatziki sauce in the pockets.
3. Top with grilled salmon fillets, mixed greens, cucumber, tomato, and red onion and serve.
4. Serve the pita pockets folded.

Nutritional Information (per serving):

Calories: Approximately 350 Protein: 35g Carbohydrates: 30g Fiber: 6g Fat: 10g Potassium: 620mg Phosphorus: 290mg Sodium: 250mg

Egg Fried Rice

Preparation Time: 20 minutes
Servings: 4

Ingredients:

- 2 cups cooked brown rice (low-phosphorus)
- 4 large eggs, lightly beaten
- 1/2 cup mixed vegetables (peas, carrots, corn)
- 1/4 cup low-sodium soy sauce
- 2 green onions, thinly sliced
- 1 tablespoon vegetable oil

Preparation:

1. Warm up the vegetable oil in a large pan or wok over medium-high heat.
2. Pour in the beaten eggs and scramble in the pan.
3. Pour in the mixed veggies and cook until tender.
4. Pour and stir in the cooked brown rice and the low-sodium soy sauce.
5. Cook, stirring constantly, until everything is cooked thoroughly.
6. Top with diced green onions.
7. Serve and enjoy your meal.

Nutritional Information (per serving):

Calories: Approximately 270 Protein: 12g Carbohydrates: 38g Fiber:3g Fat:8g Potassium:240mg Phosphorus: 150mg Sodium: 330mg

Green Curry Vegetable Soup

Preparation Time: 35 minutes
Servings: 4

Ingredients:

- 1 tablespoon green curry paste (low-sodium)

- 1 can (14 ounces) coconut milk (low-fat)
- 4 cups vegetable broth (low-sodium)
- Two measuring cups of variety of vegetables such as zucchini, bell peppers and snap peas
- 1 cup tofu, cubed
- 1 tablespoon fish sauce (optional)
- Fresh basil leaves for garnish

Preparation:

1. Heat the green curry paste in a large saucepan over a medium-low flame.
2. Stir in the coconut milk until mixed.
3. Add the vegetable broth, mixed veggies, tofu, and fish sauce (if using).
4. Cook until the veggies are soft.
5. Top with fresh basil leaves and serve.

Nutritional Information (per serving):

Calories: Approximately 220 Protein: 6g Carbohydrates: 16g Fiber: 4g Fat: 16g Potassium: 450mg Phosphorus: 100mg Sodium: 280mg

CHAPTER 5

Dinner Recipes

Dinner is more than just a meal; it is the last nourishment your body receives before going to bed. Creating pleasant and kidney-friendly dinners can have a substantial influence on overall well-being, including sleep quality, in people with CKD Stage 5. In this chapter, we will discuss the necessity of a hearty evening meal and give you a variety of delectable dishes to meet your dietary requirements.

The Importance of a Satisfying Dinner

A filling meal not only fills your stomach but also prepares your body for a night of restorative sleep. The appropriate nutrition may help you recharge, repair tissues, and sustain general health.

Kidney-Friendly Dinner Guidelines

1. **Protein and lean options:** Choose lean foods like chicken or fish that are low in phosphate and potassium.
2. **Incorporate Vegetables:** A range of colourful, low-potassium and low-phosphorus veggies can deliver critical vitamins and minerals.

3. **Mindful Seasonings:** To add flavour without using too much salt, use herbs, spices, and low-sodium seasonings.

Recipes:

Creamy Mustard Chicken

Preparation Time: 30 minutes

Servings: 4

Ingredients:

- 4 boneless, skinless chicken breasts
- 1 tablespoon olive oil
- 2 cloves garlic, minced
- 1 cup low-sodium chicken broth
- 1/2 cup low-fat Greek yogurt
- 2 tablespoons Dijon mustard
- Fresh thyme for garnish
- Salt and pepper to taste

Preparation:

1. Heat olive oil in a large pan over a medium-high flame.
2. Season the chicken breasts with salt & pepper and fry until it browns on both sides.
3. Take the chicken from the skillet and put it aside.

4. In the exact skillet, combine minced garlic, chicken broth, low-fat Greek yoghurt, and Dijon mustard. Whisk everything together until smooth.
5. Take back the chicken to the skillet and heat until it is cooked through and the sauce has solidified.
6. Top with fresh thyme before serving.

Nutritional Information (per serving):

Calories: Approximately 220 Protein: 30g Carbohydrates: 5g

Fibre: 0g Fat: 8g Potassium: 330mg Phosphorus: 250mg Sodium: 300mg

Classic Lasagna

Preparation Time: 1 hour

Servings: 6

Ingredients:

- 9 lasagna noodles (low-phosphorus)
- 1 pound lean ground beef or turkey
- 1 onion, chopped
- 2 cloves garlic, minced
- 1 can (14 ounces) low-sodium tomato sauce
- 1 can (14 ounces) low-sodium diced tomatoes
- 1 teaspoon dried basil

- 1 teaspoon dried oregano
- 1 cup low-fat ricotta cheese
- 1 cup low-fat mozzarella cheese, shredded
- 1/4 cup Parmesan cheese, grated
- Salt and pepper to taste

Preparation:

1. Cook the lasagna noodles following the packaging directions, then rinse and strain.
2. Brown the ground beef or turkey, chopped onion, and minced garlic in a pan.
3. Combine the tomato sauce, chopped tomatoes, dry basil, and dried oregano. Allow to simmer for ten minutes.
4. In a mixing dish, add the low-fat ricotta cheese, shredded mozzarella cheese, and grated Parmesan cheese.
5. In a baking dish, arrange noodles, meat sauce, and cheese mixture. Repeat the layers.
6. Bake at 350°F (175°C) for a total of thirty minutes or until bubbling and golden.
7. Serve and enjoy.

Nutritional Information (per serving):

Calories: Approximately 350 Protein: 26g Carbohydrates: 35g
Fiber: 4g Fat: 12g Potassium: 360mg Phosphorus: 220mg Sodium: 260mg

Chilli Cornbread Casserole

Preparation Time: 40 minutes

Servings: 4

Ingredients:

- 1 pound lean ground beef or turkey
- 1 onion, chopped
- 1 can (14 ounces) low-sodium kidney beans, drained and rinsed
- 1 can (14 ounces) low-sodium diced tomatoes
- 1 can (4.5 ounces) of mild green chillies
- 1 packet of low-sodium chilli seasoning mix
- 1/2 cup low-fat cornbread mix
- 1/4 cup low-fat milk
- 1 egg

Preparation:

1. Cook ground beef or turkey and chopped onion till browned in a pan.
2. Add the kidney beans, diced tomatoes, green chillies, and chilli spice. Cook for 10 minutes.
3. Combine the cornbread mix, low-fat milk, and an egg in a mixing dish.

4. Transfer the chilli mixture with the cornbread mixture in a baking dish.

5. Bake for 20 minutes at 375°F (190°C), or till the cornbread is browned and cooked through.

6. Serve and enjoy.

Nutritional Information (per serving):

Calories: Approximately 330 Protein: 26g Carbohydrates: 33g

Fiber: 6g Fat: 11g Potassium: 580mg Phosphorus: 220mg Sodium: 310mg

Sauce-less BBQ Baby Back Ribs

Preparation Time: 2 hours

Servings: 2

Ingredients:

- 1 slab of baby back ribs
- 1 tablespoon paprika
- 1 teaspoon garlic powder
- 1 teaspoon onion powder
- 1/2 teaspoon cayenne pepper (adjust to taste)
- Salt and pepper to taste

Preparation:

1. Setup the oven to 300°F (150°C).

2. Combine the paprika, garlic powder, onion powder, cayenne pepper, salt, and pepper in a small mixing bowl.

3. Massage the spice mixture all over the slab of ribs.

4. Wrap the ribs in aluminium foil and bake them for one and a half to two hours or until tender.

5. Finish on a grill for a few minutes if desired to provide a smoky taste.

6. Serve and enjoy.

Nutritional Information (per serving):

Calories: Approximately 350 Protein: 25g Carbohydrates: 2g
Fiber: 1g Fat: 26g

Chicken Pot Pie Stew

Preparation Time: 40 minutes
Servings: 4

Ingredients:

- 2 cups cooked chicken breast, diced
- 1 cup mixed vegetables (carrots, peas, corn)
- 1/4 cup onion, chopped
- 1/4 cup low-fat milk

- 1/4 cup low-sodium chicken broth
- 2 tablespoons all-purpose flour
- 1 teaspoon dried thyme
- Salt and pepper to taste

Preparation:

1. Cooked chicken, mixed veggies, chopped onion, dried thyme, salt, and pepper should all be combined in a saucepan.
2. Whisk together low-fat milk, low-sodium chicken broth, and all-purpose flour in a separate basin.
3. Pour the milk mixture over the chicken and veggies in the saucepan.
4. Cook for a total of twenty minutes or until the stew thickens.
5. Serve and enjoy the chicken pot pie stew.

Nutritional Information (per serving):

Calories: Approximately 280 Protein: 28g Carbohydrates: 20g
Fiber: 3g Fat: 10g Potassium: 450mg Phosphorus: 280mg Sodium: 210mg

Herb-crusted Roast Leg of Lamb

Preparation Time: 1 hour and 30 minutes

Servings: 4

Ingredients:

- 2 pounds of boneless leg of lamb
- 2 cloves garlic, minced
- 2 tablespoons fresh rosemary, chopped
- 2 tablespoons fresh thyme, chopped
- 1 tablespoon olive oil
- Salt and pepper to taste

Preparation:

1. Set up the oven to 350°F (175°C).
2. Using a small bowl, add minced garlic, fresh rosemary, fresh thyme, olive oil, salt, and pepper and combine.
3. Massage the herb mixture all over the leg of the lamb.
4. Roast for one hour and fifteen minutes, or until the lamb is done to your liking.
5. Serve and enjoy.

Nutritional Information (per serving):

Calories: Approximately 280 Protein: 35g Carbohydrates: 1g
Fibre: 0g Fat: 14g Potassium: 400mg Phosphorus: 230mg Sodium:
120mg

Black Bean Burger and Cilantro Slaw

Preparation Time: 30 minutes

Servings: 4

Ingredients:

- 1 can (15 ounces) low-sodium black beans, drained and
  rinsed
- 1/2 cup breadcrumbs
- 1/4 cup onion, chopped
- 1 clove garlic, minced
- 1 teaspoon cumin
- 1/2 teaspoon chilli powder (adjust to taste)
- 4 whole-grain burger buns
- 1 cup cabbage, shredded
- 1/4 cup low-fat mayonnaise
- 1/4 cup fresh cilantro, chopped
- Salt and pepper to taste

Preparation:

1. Combine the black beans, breadcrumbs, diced onion, minced garlic, cumin, and chilli powder in a food processor. Blend until everything is properly blended.
2. Form the bean mixture into four patties and grill or cook on the stovetop until cooked through and slightly crisped.
3. To make the slaw, mix shredded cabbage, low-fat mayonnaise, fresh cilantro, salt, and pepper in a mixing dish.
4. Serve the black bean burgers with a cilantro slaw on whole-grain buns.

Nutritional Information (per serving):

Calories: Approximately 280 Protein: 12g Carbohydrates: 50g
Fiber: 8g Fat: 4g Potassium: 390mg Phosphorus: 150mg Sodium: 320mg

Spaghetti and Asparagus Carbonara

Preparation Time: 30 minutes

Servings: 4

Ingredients:

- 8 ounces whole-wheat spaghetti (low-phosphorus)
- One bunch of trimmed and chopped asparagus
- 2 large eggs
- 1/2 cup Parmesan cheese, grated
- 1/4 cup low-fat milk
- 4 slices low-sodium bacon, cooked and crumbled
- Salt and black pepper to taste

Preparation:

1. Prepare the whole-wheat spaghetti according to package guidelines, adding asparagus for the final 3 minutes.
2. Whisk together big eggs, grated Parmesan cheese, low-fat milk, and cooked, crumbled bacon in a mixing bowl.
3. Return the pasta and asparagus to the saucepan after draining.
4. Stir together the egg and cheese mixture with the hot pasta. The heat will cook the eggs, resulting in a creamy sauce.
5. Adjust the seasoning using salt and pepper to taste.
6. Serve and enjoy.

Nutritional Information (per serving):

Calories: Approximately 350 Protein: 20g Carbohydrates: 50g Fiber: 8g Fat: 10g Potassium: 400mg Phosphorus: 160mg Sodium: 300mg

Vegan Thai Cucumber Salad

Preparation Time: 20 minutes

Servings: 4

Ingredients:

- 4 cucumbers, sliced
- 1 red onion, thinly sliced
- 1/4 cup fresh cilantro, chopped
- 1/4 cup fresh mint, chopped
- 1/4 cup rice vinegar (low-sodium)
- 2 tablespoons low-sodium soy sauce
- 1 tablespoon agave syrup
- A half-teaspoon of red pepper flakes

Preparation:

1. Add the sliced cucumbers, thinly sliced red onion, cilantro, and mint in a large mixing dish.
2. In a separate dish, combine rice vinegar, low-sodium soy sauce, agave syrup, and red pepper flakes and whisk.

3. Transfer the dressing to the cucumber salad and toss.

4. Serve and enjoy.

Nutritional Information (per serving):

Calories: Approximately 80 Protein: 2g Carbohydrates: 18g

Fiber: 3g Fat: 0g Potassium: 330mg Phosphorus: 50mg Sodium: 160mg

Grilled Fish Tacos

Preparation Time: 30 minutes

Servings: 4

Ingredients:

- 4 white fish fillets (e.g., tilapia or cod)
- 1 tablespoon olive oil
- 1 teaspoon cumin
- 1 teaspoon chilli powder (adjust to taste)
- 8 small whole-grain tortillas
- 1 cup red cabbage, shredded
- 1 cup low-fat Greek yogurt
- 1 lime, juiced
- 1/4 cup fresh cilantro, chopped
- Salt and pepper to taste

Preparation:

1. Set the grill to medium-high.
2. In a small dish, mix the olive oil, cumin, chilli powder, salt, and pepper. Smear the fish fillets with the mixture.
3. Grill the fish fillets for three to four minutes on each side, or until cooked thoroughly and have grill marks.
4. In a separate dish, add the shredded red cabbage, low-fat Greek yoghurt, lime juice, and chopped cilantro. Adjust the seasoning with salt and pepper as preferred.
5. Heat the whole-grain tortillas on the grill for about a minute on each of the sides.
6. Assemble your fish tacos by layering warmed tortillas with grilled fish, cabbage slaw, and more cilantro.
7. Serve and enjoy.

Nutritional Information (per serving):

Calories: Approximately 250 Protein: 25g Carbohydrates: 30g
Fiber: 5g Fat: 6g Potassium: 350mg Phosphorus: 200mg Sodium: 200mg

CHAPTER 6

Smart snacking is an important part of controlling CKD Stage 5. Whether you have a mid-morning need or need an energy boost in the afternoon, choosing the correct snacks may make a significant impact on your overall well-being. In this chapter, we'll look at the function of snacks in CKD management and provide you with a variety of kidney-friendly snack alternatives that are both nutritional and gratifying.

The Role of Snacks in CKD Management.

Snacks play an important part in your dietary management, helping to maintain energy levels, keep hunger at bay, and meet your nutritional needs. By choosing the correct snacks, you may guarantee that your daily nutritional needs are satisfied without jeopardizing your kidney health.

Kidney-Friendly Snacking Strategies

1. **Balanced Options:** Choose snacks with a variety of nutrients, such as protein, fibre, and healthy fats.
2. **Portion Control:** Watch your portion sizes to prevent consuming too much potassium and phosphorus.

3. **Low-Sodium Snacks:** Choose low-sodium snacks to help regulate your blood pressure and renal function.

Recipes:

Homemade Herbed Biscuits

Preparation Time: 30 minutes

Servings: 6

Ingredients:
- 1 cup all-purpose flour
- 1 teaspoon baking powder
- 1/4 teaspoon salt
- 1/4 teaspoon dried thyme
- 1/4 teaspoon dried rosemary
- 1/4 teaspoon dried basil
- 1/4 cup low-fat buttermilk
- 2 tablespoons unsalted butter, melted

Preparation:
1. Set the oven temperature to 425°F (220°C).
2. Combine the all-purpose flour, baking powder, salt, dried thyme, dried rosemary, and dried basil in a mixing dish.

3. Add in the low-fat buttermilk and the melted unsalted butter and mix till a dough forms.
4. Put spoonfuls of dough on a baking sheet and bake for 10-12 minutes, till it's golden brown.
5. Serve and enjoy your delicious snack

Nutritional Information (per serving):

Calories: Approximately 130 Protein: 2g Carbohydrates: 16g Fiber: 1g Fat: 6g Potassium: 45mg Phosphorus: 65mg Sodium: 190mg

Very Berry Bread Pudding

Preparation Time: 45 minutes

Servings: 4

Ingredients:
- 2 cups whole-grain bread cubes
- One half cup of a variety of berries like blueberries, strawberries and raspberries
- 1 cup low-fat milk
- 2 large eggs
- 1/4 cup agave syrup
- 1/2 teaspoon vanilla extract
- 1/4 teaspoon cinnamon
- 1/4 teaspoon nutmeg

Preparation:

1. Set up the oven to 350°F (175°C).
2. Combine whole-grain bread pieces and mixed berries in a container.
3. In another dish, combine low-fat milk, big eggs, agave syrup, vanilla essence, cinnamon, and nutmeg.
4. Spread the milk mixture over the bread and berries, making sure that all of the bread cubes are submerged.
5. Bake for thirty to thirty-five until the pudding is set and its top is brown.
6. Serve and enjoy.

Nutritional Information (per serving):

Calories: Approximately 220 Protein: 7g Carbohydrates: 38g
Fiber: 4g Fat: 5g Potassium: 250mg Phosphorus: 200mg Sodium: 180mg

Orange and Cinnamon Biscotti

Preparation Time: 1 hour and 15 minutes
Servings: 10

Ingredients:

- 1 1/2 cups all-purpose flour
- 1/2 cup sugar

- 1/2 teaspoon baking powder
- 1/4 teaspoon salt
- 2 large eggs
- 1 teaspoon orange zest
- 1/2 teaspoon ground cinnamon

Preparation:

1. Set the temperature of the oven to 350°F/175°C.
2. Combine the all-purpose flour, sugar, baking powder, and salt in a mixing container.
3. Whisk together the big eggs, orange zest, and ground cinnamon in a separate container.
4. Stir in the egg mixture and dry ingredients up until a dough forms.
5. Bake for 25-30 minutes, or until the dough is slightly brown.
6. Allow the log to cool for a few minutes after removing it from the oven. Then cut it into biscotti and bake for another ten to fifteen minutes, or until crisp.
7. Savour and enjoy.

Nutritional Information (per serving):

Calories: Approximately 130 Protein: 3g Carbohydrates: 26g

Fiber: 1g Fat: 2g Potassium: 45mg Phosphorus: 40mg Sodium: 50mg

Sweet and Nutty Protein Bars

Preparation Time: 20 minutes

Servings: 8

Ingredients:

- 1 cup rolled oats
- 1/2 cup almonds, chopped
- 1/2 cup dates, pitted and chopped
- 1/4 cup almond butter
- 2 tablespoons honey
- 1/2 teaspoon vanilla extract
- 1/4 teaspoon salt

Preparation:

1. Combine the rolled oats, chopped almonds, chopped dates, almond butter, honey, vanilla essence, and salt in a food processor.
2. Process the ingredients until they come together and become sticky.

3. Refrigerate for about 2 hours after pressing the mixture into a square baking dish.
4. Slice into bars and serve.

Nutritional Information (per serving):

Calories: Approximately 180 Protein: 4g Carbohydrates: 25g Fiber: 3g Fat: 8g Potassium: 180mg Phosphorus: 70mg Sodium: 50mg

Curried Cashews

Preparation Time: 15 minutes

Servings: 4

Ingredients:
- 2 cups cashews
- 1 tablespoon olive oil
- 1 teaspoon curry powder (adjust to taste)
- 1/4 teaspoon salt

Preparation:
1. In a medium heat flame, using a skillet, heat the olive oil.
2. Add and Sauté the cashews and curry powder until they are toasted and covered with the curry mix.
3. Take from heat and season with salt. Let it cool down before serving.

Nutritional Information (per serving):

Calories: Approximately 220 Protein: 5g Carbohydrates: 12g Fiber: 2g Fat: 17g Potassium: 240mg Phosphorus: 150mg Sodium: 70mg

Strawberry and Chocolate Frozen Yogurt Bark

Preparation Time: 2 hours

Servings: 4

Ingredients:

- 2 cups low-fat Greek yogurt
- 1/4 cup dark chocolate chips (low-phosphorus)
- 1/2 cup strawberries, sliced
- 2 tablespoons honey
- 1/4 teaspoon vanilla extract

Preparation:

1. In a mixing dish, add low-fat Greek yoghurt, dark chocolate chips, honey, and vanilla extract.
2. Line a baking sheet with some parchment paper and spread the mixture out.
3. Sprinkle strawberries that have been on top of the yoghurt.
4. Freeze for about two hours at a time or until completely solid.
5. Divide into pieces and serve.

Nutritional Information (per serving):

Calories: Approximately 180 Protein: 7g Carbohydrates: 25g Fiber: 2g Fat: 6g Potassium: 270mg Phosphorus: 100mg Sodium: 50mg

Carrot Cake Energy Bites

Preparation Time: 20 minutes

Servings: 8

Ingredients:

- 1 cup carrots, grated
- 1 cup rolled oats
- 1/2 cup unsweetened shredded coconut
- 1/4 cup almond butter
- 1/4 cup honey
- 1/2 teaspoon ground cinnamon
- 1/4 teaspoon nutmeg

Preparation:

1. In a mixing dish, add grated carrots, rolled oats, unsweetened shredded coconut, almond butter, honey, crushed cinnamon, and nutmeg.
2. Mix until completely blended.

3. Shape it into little energy bits and refrigerate till it becomes hard.

Nutritional Information (per serving):

Calories: Approximately 140 Protein: 3g Carbohydrates: 18g Fiber: 2g Fat: 7g Potassium: 170mg Phosphorus: 60mg Sodium: 20mg

Cheesy Popcorn

Preparation Time: 5 minutes

Servings: 2

Ingredients:

- 4 cups air-popped popcorn
- 2 tablespoons nutritional yeast
- 1/2 teaspoon garlic powder
- 1/4 teaspoon onion powder
- Salt to taste

Preparation:

1. Begin by air-popping 4 cups of popcorn. You may pop the popcorn using an air popper or your favourite technique.
2. In a large mixing dish, combine the air-popped popcorn.

3. Add 2 teaspoons of nutritional yeast to the popcorn. Nutritional yeast will give the popcorn a cheesy taste without using real cheese.

4. Add 1/2 teaspoon garlic powder for a delicious, garlicky flavour.

5. To improve the taste, add 1/4 teaspoon onion powder.

6. Season the mixture with salt to taste. Start with a small quantity of salt and add more as desired.

7. Toss the popcorn with the ingredients in a mixing basin until equally covered with the nutritional yeast, garlic powder, onion powder, and salt.

8. Your Cheesy Popcorn is now ready to serve as a tasty and healthier alternative to typical cheese popcorn.

9. Serve immediately, and feel free to modify the spices to your liking.

Nutritional Information (per serving):
Calories: Approximately 80 Protein: 3g Carbohydrates: 13g

Fiber: 3g Fat: 2g Potassium: 70mg Phosphorus: 80mg Sodium: 190mg

Maple Granola

Preparation Time: 30 minutes

Servings: 10

Ingredients:

- 2 cups old-fashioned rolled oats
- 1/2 cup chopped almonds
- 1/4 cup chopped walnuts
- 1/4 cup chopped pecans
- 1/4 cup pure maple syrup
- 2 tablespoons vegetable oil
- 1/2 teaspoon ground cinnamon
- 1/4 teaspoon salt

Preparation:

1. Set the oven temperature to 325°F (165°C).
2. Combine old-fashioned rolled oats, chopped almonds, chopped walnuts, chopped pecans, pure maple syrup, vegetable oil, cinnamon, and salt in a large mixing bowl.
3. Transfer the mixture to a baking sheet and Bake for twenty to twenty-five minutes, stirring regularly, until golden brown.
4. Serve and enjoy.

Nutritional Information (per serving):

Calories: Approximately 160 Protein: 4g Carbohydrates: 15g
Fiber: 2g Fat: 10g Potassium: 150mg Phosphorus: 90mg Sodium:
50mg

Zucchini Fritters with Dill Yogurt

Preparation Time: 30 minutes
Servings: 4

Ingredients:

- 2 zucchinis, grated
- 1/4 cup whole-wheat flour
- 1/4 cup grated Parmesan cheese
- 1/4 cup fresh dill, chopped
- 1 large egg
- 1/4 cup low-fat Greek yogurt
- 1 tablespoon lemon juice
- 1 clove garlic, minced
- Salt and pepper to taste

Preparation:

1. Place the shredded zucchini in a clean kitchen towel and squeeze out any excess liquid.

2. In a mixing dish, add grated zucchini, whole-wheat flour, grated Parmesan cheese, fresh dill, and a large egg. Mix until completely blended.

3. Warm a skillet with a tiny quantity of oil over medium-high heat.

4. To prepare fritters, spoon the zucchini mixture into a pan. Cook for about 2-3 minutes on both sides, until it becomes golden brown.

5. To prepare a dipping sauce, whisk together low-fat Greek yoghurt, lemon juice, minced garlic, salt, and pepper in a separate bowl.

6. Serve the zucchini fritters alongside the dill yoghurt sauce.

Nutritional Information (per serving):

Calories: Approximately 120 Protein: 7g Carbohydrates: 11g

Fiber: 2g Fat: 6g Potassium: 350mg Phosphorus: 130mg Sodium: 170mg

Pineapple Smoothie

Preparation Time: 10 minutes

Servings: 2

Ingredients:

- 1 cup fresh pineapple chunks
- 1/2 cup low-fat Greek yogurt
- 1/2 cup unsweetened almond milk
- 1/2 teaspoon honey (optional)
- 1/4 teaspoon ground ginger
- Ice cubes (optional)

Preparation:

1. Blend fresh pineapple chunks, low-fat Greek yoghurt, unsweetened almond milk, honey (if used), and ground ginger in a blender.
2. Blend until the mixture is smooth.
3. If you like a cooler smoothie, add some ice cubes.

Nutritional Information (per serving):

Calories: Approximately 90 Protein: 5g Carbohydrates: 15g

Fiber: 2g Fat: 1g Potassium: 170mg Phosphorus: 85mg Sodium: 50mg

CHAPTER 7

Dessert Recipes

It may seem difficult to satisfy your sweet taste while controlling CKD Stage 5, but it is not impossible. In this chapter, we'll look at how to enjoy tasty sweets while adhering to kidney-friendly dietary guidelines. From fruity pleasures to creamy creations, you'll find inventive ways to indulge in sweets without jeopardizing your health.

Individuals with CKD, like everyone else, have times when they need something sweet. You may still enjoy delectable sweets while keeping your kidney health in check if you know how to manage sugary delights.

Kid-Friendly Dessert Essential

1. **Low-Phosphorus Alternatives:** Learn how to choose phosphorus-free products and recipes, which is critical for CKD treatment.
2. **Sweeteners and substitutions:** Look for sweeteners and substitutions that are good for kidney-friendly desserts.
3. **Portion Control:** Understand the significance of portion control while eating sweets.

Recipes:

Dried Cranberry Fruit Bars

Preparation Time: 20 minutes

Servings: 8

Ingredients:

- 1 cup dried cranberries (low-phosphorus)
- 1/2 cup rolled oats
- 1/4 cup unsweetened applesauce
- 1/4 cup almond butter
- 1/4 teaspoon ground cinnamon

Preparation:

1. Combine the dried cranberries, rolled oats, unsweetened applesauce, almond butter, and ground cinnamon in a food processor.
2. Blend until the mixture is smooth.
3. Press the mixture into a square baking dish and refrigerate until hard.
4. Slice and serve in bars.

Nutritional Information (per serving):

Calories: Approximately 100 Protein: 2g Carbohydrates: 18g Fiber: 3g Fat: 4g Potassium: 90mg Phosphorus: 45mg Sodium: 0mg

Chewy Lemon-Ginger-Coconut Cookies

Preparation Time: 30 minutes

Servings: 12

Ingredients:

- 1 cup unsweetened shredded coconut
- 1/2 cup almond flour
- 2 tablespoons honey
- 1 tablespoon lemon zest
- 1/2 teaspoon ground ginger
- 1/4 teaspoon vanilla extract
- 1 large egg

Preparation:

1. Set up the oven to 350°F (175°C) and cover a baking sheet with sheets of parchment paper.
2. In a mixing dish, add unsweetened shredded coconut, almond flour, honey, lemon zest, crushed ginger, and vanilla essence.

3. Mix in the beaten egg until a dough forms.

4. Pour spoonfuls of dough onto the baking sheet and flatten with a fork.

5. Bake for twelve to fifteen minutes, or until the cookies are brown.

Nutritional Information (per serving):

Calories: Approximately 100 Protein: 2g Carbohydrates: 8g

Fiber: 3g Fat: 7g Potassium: 85mg Phosphorus: 35mg Sodium: 10mg

Molten Mint Chocolate Brownie

Preparation Time: 40 minutes

Servings: 4

Ingredients:

- 1/2 cup unsweetened cocoa powder
- 1/4 cup almond flour
- 1/4 cup honey
- 1/4 teaspoon mint extract
- 1/4 teaspoon vanilla extract
- 2 large eggs
- 1/4 cup dark chocolate chips (low-phosphorus)

Preparation:

1. Set up the oven to 350°F (175°C) and coat a baking dish with cooking spray.

2. Unsweetened cocoa powder, almond flour, honey, mint essence, vanilla extract, and beaten eggs should all be combined in a mixing dish.

3. Mix in dark chocolate chips.

4. Transfer the mixture to a baking dish and bake for 20-25 minutes, or until the edges of the pan are set but the middle is still somewhat molten.

5. Wait for a few minutes of cooling down before serving.

Nutritional Information (per serving):

Calories: Approximately 200 Protein: 5g Carbohydrates: 25g

Fiber: 5g Fat: 10g Potassium: 200mg Phosphorus: 80mg Sodium: 30mg

Sunburst Lemon Bars

Preparation Time: 45 minutes

Servings: 8

Ingredients:

- 1 cup almond flour
- 1/4 cup honey
- 1/4 cup lemon juice
- 1 tablespoon lemon zest
- 1/2 teaspoon vanilla extract
- 2 large eggs

Preparation:

1. Set up the oven to 350°F (175°C) and prepare a baking dish using sheets of parchment paper.
2. In a mixing dish, add almond flour, honey, lemon juice, lemon zest, and vanilla essence.
3. Mix in the beaten eggs until well mixed.
4. Transfer the mixture to the baking dish and bake for 20-25 minutes, up until the bars are set.
5. Allow to cool down before dicing into bars.

Nutritional Information (per serving):

Calories: Approximately 120 Protein: 4g Carbohydrates: 12g Fiber: 2g Fat: 7g Potassium: 80mg Phosphorus: 50mg Sodium: 20mg

Cherry Sorbet

Preparation Time: 10 minutes (plus freezing time)

Servings: 4

Ingredients:

- 2 cups frozen cherries
- 1/4 cup water
- 1/4 cup honey
- 1 teaspoon lemon juice

Preparation:

1. Blend frozen cherries, water, honey, and lemon juice in a blender.
2. Blend until completely smooth.
3. Transfer the mixture into a freezer-safe container and freeze for approximately 2-3 hours, or until the sorbet is solid.
4. Scoop and serve.

Nutritional Information (per serving):

Calories: Approximately 100 Protein: 1g Carbohydrates: 25g

Fiber: 3g Fat: 0.5g Potassium: 170mg Phosphorus: 30mg Sodium: 0mg

Caramel Apples

Preparation Time: 20 minutes

Servings: 4

Ingredients:

- 4 small apples
- 1/4 cup low-sugar caramel sauce (low-phosphorus)
- 1/4 cup chopped nuts (e.g., pecans, almonds)

Preparation:

1. The apples should be washed and dried.
2. Insert skewers or popsicle sticks into the apples.
3. Dip each apple in the sugar-free caramel sauce.
4. Roll chopped nuts over the caramel-covered apples.
5. Before serving, let them cool and solidify.

Nutritional Information (per serving):

Calories: Approximately 150 Protein: 1g Carbohydrates: 30g
Fiber: 4g Fat: 4g Potassium: 200mg Phosphorus: 40mg Sodium: 30mg

Chocolate Coconut Macaroons

Preparation Time: 30 minutes

Servings: 12

Ingredients:

- 2 cups unsweetened shredded coconut
- 1/4 cup unsweetened cocoa powder
- 1/4 cup honey
- 1/4 cup almond flour
- 1/4 teaspoon vanilla extract
- 2 large egg whites

Preparation:

1. Turn up the oven to 350°F (175°C) and line a baking sheet with sheets of parchment paper.
2. In a mixing bowl, add unsweetened shredded coconut, unsweetened cocoa powder, honey, almond flour, and vanilla extract.
3. In another separate dish, beat the egg whites until firm peaks form.
4. Gently incorporate the beaten egg whites into the coconut mixture until thoroughly mixed.
5. Transfer spoonfuls of the mixture onto the prepared baking sheet.

6. Bake for fifteen to twenty minutes, till the macaroons are gently browned.

Nutritional Information (per serving):

Calories: Approximately 100 Protein: 2g Carbohydrates: 10g Fiber: 3g Fat: 6g Potassium: 75mg Phosphorus: 35mg Sodium: 20mg

Blueberry Squares

Preparation Time: 35 minutes

Servings: 8

Ingredients:

- 1 cup almond flour
- 1/4 cup honey
- 1/4 cup unsweetened applesauce
- 1/2 teaspoon lemon zest
- 1 cup fresh or frozen blueberries

Preparation:

1. Set up the oven to 350°F (175°C) and prepare a baking dish lined with parchment paper.
2. In a mixing dish, add and combine almond flour, honey, unsweetened applesauce, and lemon zest.

3. Distribute half of the mixture to the bottom of the baking dish.

4. Spread the blueberries equally over the mixture.

5. Scatter the remainder of the almond flour mixture on top.

6. Bake for twenty to twenty-five or until the top is brown and the blueberries are bubbling.

Nutritional Information (per serving):

Calories: Approximately 120 Protein: 2g Carbohydrates: 14g

Fiber: 2g Fat: 7g Potassium: 70mg Phosphorus: 40mg Sodium: 10mg

Mini Pecan Pies

Preparation Time: 35 minutes

Servings: 8

Ingredients:

- 1 cup chopped pecans
- 1/4 cup almond flour
- 1/4 cup honey
- 1/4 cup unsweetened applesauce
- 1/4 teaspoon vanilla extract
- 2 large eggs

Preparation:

1. Turn up the oven to 350°F (175°C) and cover a muffin pan with paper muffin liners.

2. Add the chopped pecans, almond flour, honey, unsweetened applesauce, and vanilla extract in a mixing dish.

3. Add the beaten eggs to the mixture. Mix it up together until everything is incorporated.

4. Distribute the mixture among the muffin cups equally.

5. Bake the pies for approximately fifteen to twenty minutes, or until they are firm and slightly browned.

Nutritional Information (per serving):

Calories: Approximately 130 Protein: 3g Carbohydrates: 12g

Fiber: 2g Fat: 8g Potassium: 70mg Phosphorus: 40mg Sodium: 15mg

Watermelon Fruit Pizza

Preparation Time: 20 minutes

Servings: 6

Ingredients:

- 1/2 small watermelon, sliced into rounds
- 1 cup low-fat Greek yogurt
- 1/4 cup mixed berries (e.g., strawberries, blueberries)
- 1/4 cup kiwi, sliced
- 1/4 cup unsweetened shredded coconut

Preparation:

1. Watermelon should be cut into rounds to make "pizza crusts."
2. Cover each watermelon round with a coating of low-fat Greek yoghurt.
3. Garnish with kiwi slices and unsweetened shredded coconut.
4. Cut and serve in wedges.

Nutritional Information (per serving):

Calories: Approximately 90 Protein: 4g Carbohydrates: 15g

Fiber: 2g Fat: 2g Potassium: 220mg Phosphorus: 60mg Sodium: 20mg

CHAPTER 8

Planning Kidney-Friendly Meals for the Week

Meal planning is an important part of treating CKD Stage 5 because it helps you consume a balanced meal while following dietary restrictions. Here's a step-by-step method for planning kidney-friendly meals for the week:

1.Be aware of your dietary restrictions: Before you begin preparing, it's critical to understand your dietary limits, which may include potassium, phosphorus, salt, and fluid consumption restrictions. Consult your healthcare physician or a certified dietician to evaluate your requirements.

2. Establish Realistic Objectives: Define your nutritional objectives, such as lowering potassium consumption or managing phosphorus intake. Understanding your goals can help you plan meals.

3. Make a Weekly plan: Begin by making a weekly plan including your breakfast, lunch, supper, and snack choices. Consider integrating a variety of meals to ensure you're receiving a broad range of nutrients.

4. Select Kidney-Friendly Ingredients: Choose components that are low in potassium, phosphorus, and salt. Fresh, unprocessed meals are often lower in these minerals than processed foods.

5. Balance Macronutrients: Make sure your meals include a good mix of carbs, protein, and healthy fats. It is best to include lean protein, nutritious carbohydrates, and lots of fruits and vegetables.

6. Portion Control: Pay strict attention to portion sizes. Use measuring cups and scales as required to remain within the suggested serving sizes. This is especially crucial for nutrients like grains and proteins.

7. Plan for Variety: Variety is important not just for taste but also for getting a broad range of nutrients. To minimize meal boredom, switch up your protein sources, veggies, and grains.

8. Pre-Prep items: Consider pre-prepping certain items to make cooking over the week more convenient. For example, wash and slice veggies or divide out snacks.

9. Balance Nutrients in Meals: Strive for nutritional balance in each meal. A typical dish would contain a lean protein source (e.g., chicken or tofu), a side of low-phosphorus grains (e.g., rice or quinoa), and a selection of cooked or raw low-potassium veggies (e.g., green beans, carrots, or bell peppers).

10. Monitor Fluid Intake: Keep an eye on your fluid intake, particularly if you have stringent fluid limits. You may need to minimize drinks during meals and opt for alternatives such as sucking on ice chips.

11. Include Snacks: Healthy, kidney-friendly snacks may help decrease appetite between meals. Choose from fresh fruit, unsalted rice cakes, or low-phosphorus yoghurt.

12. Review and Adjust: After a week, evaluate how well your food plan worked for you. Did you reach your nutritional targets? Were the portion sizes appropriate? Make any necessary revisions for the next week.

Meal planning for CKD Stage 5 may seem daunting at first, but with repetition, it becomes more intuitive. Remember that it's important to work with a healthcare professional or registered dietitian to develop a meal plan that's personalized to your specific requirements. By following these steps and being consistent, you may better manage your kidney health via intelligent, kidney-friendly meal planning.

Strategies For Portion Control

Portion control is a critical component of CKD Stage 5 management. It ensures that you ingest the appropriate quantities of nutrients and prevents overloading your body with chemicals such as potassium and phosphorus. Here are some excellent ways to control your portion sizes while still enjoying your meals:

1. Use Measuring Tools: Purchase measuring cups and a kitchen scale. These tools may assist you in precisely portioning items such as cereals, proteins, and snacks. Understanding what a genuine serving size looks like is quite useful.

2. Plate Method: The plate approach is imagining your plate split into portions. Half of your plate should include non-starchy veggies (poor in potassium), one-quarter lean protein (e.g., chicken, fish), and one-quarter grains or starches (low-phosphorus alternatives). This strategy not only limits portions but also promotes balanced eating.

3. Single Servings: Whenever feasible, buy meals in single-serving packaging. This removes the need to measure and makes portion management easier. Choose pre-packaged snacks or individually portioned frozen veggies.

4. Read Food Labels: Pay strict attention to food labels. Check serving sizes and nutritional information to ensure you're eating quantities that adhere to your dietary limitations. Keep a watch on potassium, phosphorus, and sodium levels.

5. Avoid Family-Style Serving: When eating with guests, it is customary to set serving dishes on the table for everyone to assist themselves. Instead, serve portioned meals from the kitchen to avoid overeating. This also decreases the urge to have seconds.

6. Pre-Portion Snacks: Divide snacks into portion-controlled containers. This makes it simpler to grab a single serving of nuts, apples, or other snacks without overindulging.

7. Use Smaller dishes: When serving meals, use smaller dishes. The visual illusion of a full plate might deceive your brain into feeling pleased with fewer quantities.

8. Savor Your Food: Eating attentively might help you limit your portion sizes. Slow down, eat your meal properly, and relish each mouthful. This provides your body more time to notify when it's full.

9. Stop Eating When Satisfied: Pay attention to your body's indications of hunger and fullness. Quit eating when you're satisfied, not when your plate is empty. You could always save leftovers for a little later.

10. Drink Water Before Meals: Drinking a glass of water before meals will help reduce your appetite and avoid overeating. Furthermore, keeping hydrated is critical for kidney health.

11. Track Your Consumption: Consider maintaining a food diary to track your portion sizes and nutrient consumption. This might help you discover places where your portions may need to be adjusted.

12. Seek Help: Don't be hesitant to seek help from a licensed dietitian or nutritionist who specializes in renal health. They may provide you with tailored advice on portion management and meal planning.

Remember that mastering portion control requires time and practice. Be patient with yourself and concentrate on the long-term advantages of treating your kidney health. By using these tactics, you may strike a balance between enjoying your meals and protecting your health in CKD Stage 5.

CONCLUSION

Embracing a Healthier, Kidney-Friendly Future

As we near the end of the "CKD Stage 5 Cookbook for Beginners," it's evident that the path to treating Chronic Kidney Disease (CKD) at Stage 5 is one of dedication, perseverance, and commitment. We've traversed the treacherous terrain of CKD, learning not only about the obstacles it presents but also about the powerful tools at our disposal to help us negotiate this route.

This cookbook is more than simply a compilation of dishes; it is a lighthouse for individuals dealing with CKD Stage 5. It demonstrates that eating can be both medicine and pleasure. Most significantly, it represents the extraordinary journey you've undertaken to restore your health and well-being.

The following main lessons from this book have enlightened your path:

- CKD Stage 5 is a daunting task, but with careful nutritional control, we may improve our quality of life.
- A kidney-friendly diet is an essential part of this journey, helping you to slow the advancement of the illness, manage symptoms, and maximize your overall health.

- With the help of qualified dietitians and the information on these pages, you now have the skills you need to prepare tasty, healthy meals while adhering to CKD dietary restrictions.

This book isn't the conclusion of your narrative; it's the beginning of a better, kidney-friendly future. The recipes you've found, meal plans you've devised, and portion control tactics you've adopted will allow you to enjoy life to the fullest while managing CKD.

Remember to keep your journey in mind as you flip the last page. You are not alone on this road. Reach out for help, both from healthcare experts and from a network of people who understand your difficulties. This journey is about nourishing not just your body, but also your soul, and finding pleasure in the minor successes along the road.

The chapters of your life may have changed, but they are still full of possibility, opportunity, and the ability to prepare tasty, kidney-friendly meals. With your increased understanding and dedication, welcome this future with open arms, knowing that you have the strength to prosper despite the hurdles. Here's to your health, your perseverance, and a future full of kidney-friendly treats.

BONUS

Meal Planner Journal

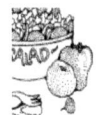 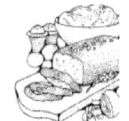

WEEKLY MEAL PLANNER

MONTH:

WEEK:

DAY	BREAKFAST	LUNCH	DINNER	SNACK
MON				
TUE				
WED				
THU				
FRI				
SAT				
SUN				

IMPORTANT NOTES

SHOPPING LIST

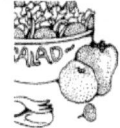
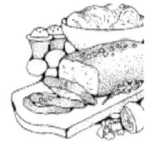

WEEKLY MEAL PLANNER

MONTH:

WEEK:

DAY	BREAKFAST	LUNCH	DINNER	SNACK
MON				
TUE				
WED				
THU				
FRI				
SAT				
SUN				

IMPORTANT NOTES

SHOPPING LIST

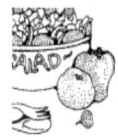 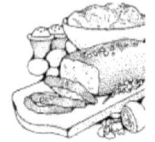

WEEKLY MEAL PLANNER

MONTH:

WEEK:

DAY	BREAKFAST	LUNCH	DINNER	SNACK
MON				
TUE				
WED				
THU				
FRI				
SAT				
SUN				

IMPORTANT NOTES

SHOPPING LIST

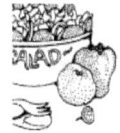
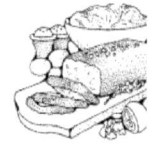

WEEKLY MEAL PLANNER

MONTH:

WEEK:

DAY	BREAKFAST	LUNCH	DINNER	SNACK
MON				
TUE				
WED				
THU				
FRI				
SAT				
SUN				

IMPORTANT NOTES

SHOPPING LIST

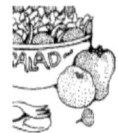 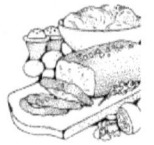

WEEKLY MEAL PLANNER

MONTH:

WEEK:

DAY	BREAKFAST	LUNCH	DINNER	SNACK
MON				
TUE				
WED				
THU				
FRI				
SAT				
SUN				

IMPORTANT NOTES

SHOPPING LIST

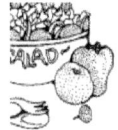 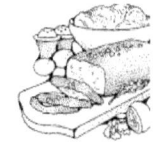

WEEKLY MEAL PLANNER

MONTH:

WEEK:

DAY	BREAKFAST	LUNCH	DINNER	SNACK
MON				
TUE				
WED				
THU				
FRI				
SAT				
SUN				

IMPORTANT NOTES

SHOPPING LIST

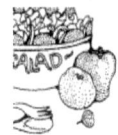 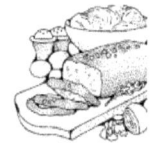

WEEKLY MEAL PLANNER

MONTH:

WEEK:

DAY	BREAKFAST	LUNCH	DINNER	SNACK
MON				
TUE				
WED				
THU				
FRI				
SAT				
SUN				

IMPORTANT NOTES

SHOPPING LIST

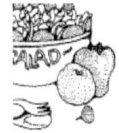 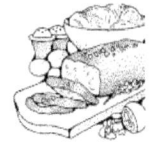

WEEKLY MEAL PLANNER

MONTH:

WEEK:

DAY	BREAKFAST	LUNCH	DINNER	SNACK
MON				
TUE				
WED				
THU				
FRI				
SAT				
SUN				

IMPORTANT NOTES

SHOPPING LIST

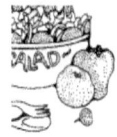 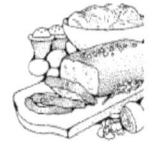

WEEKLY MEAL PLANNER

MONTH:

WEEK:

DAY	BREAKFAST	LUNCH	DINNER	SNACK
MON				
TUE				
WED				
THU				
FRI				
SAT				
SUN				

IMPORTANT NOTES

SHOPPING LIST

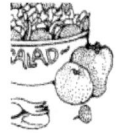 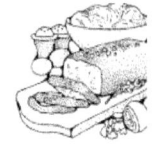

WEEKLY MEAL PLANNER

MONTH:

WEEK:

DAY	BREAKFAST	LUNCH	DINNER	SNACK
MON				
TUE				
WED				
THU				
FRI				
SAT				
SUN				

IMPORTANT NOTES

SHOPPING LIST

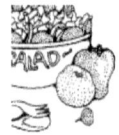
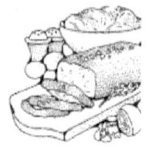

WEEKLY MEAL PLANNER

MONTH:

WEEK:

DAY	BREAKFAST	LUNCH	DINNER	SNACK
MON				
TUE				
WED				
THU				
FRI				
SAT				
SUN				

IMPORTANT NOTES

SHOPPING LIST

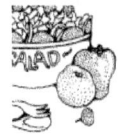 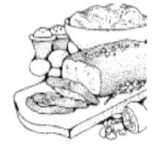

WEEKLY MEAL PLANNER

MONTH:

WEEK:

DAY	BREAKFAST	LUNCH	DINNER	SNACK
MON				
TUE				
WED				
THU				
FRI				
SAT				
SUN				

IMPORTANT NOTES

SHOPPING LIST

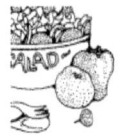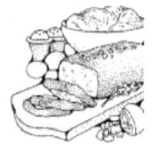

WEEKLY MEAL PLANNER

MONTH:

WEEK:

DAY	BREAKFAST	LUNCH	DINNER	SNACK
MON				
TUE				
WED				
THU				
FRI				
SAT				
SUN				

IMPORTANT NOTES

SHOPPING LIST

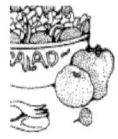 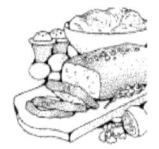

WEEKLY MEAL PLANNER

MONTH:

WEEK:

DAY	BREAKFAST	LUNCH	DINNER	SNACK
MON				
TUE				
WED				
THU				
FRI				
SAT				
SUN				

IMPORTANT NOTES

SHOPPING LIST

:

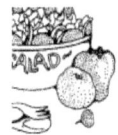 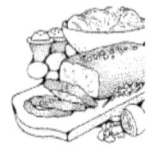

WEEKLY MEAL PLANNER

MONTH:

WEEK:

DAY	BREAKFAST	LUNCH	DINNER	SNACK
MON				
TUE				
WED				
THU				
FRI				
SAT				
SUN				

IMPORTANT NOTES

SHOPPING LIST

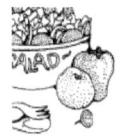 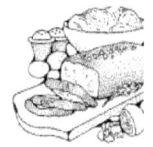

WEEKLY MEAL PLANNER

MONTH:

WEEK:

DAY	BREAKFAST	LUNCH	DINNER	SNACK
MON				
TUE				
WED				
THU				
FRI				
SAT				
SUN				

IMPORTANT NOTES

SHOPPING LIST

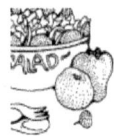 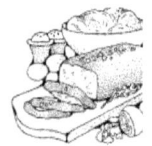

WEEKLY MEAL PLANNER

MONTH:

WEEK:

DAY	BREAKFAST	LUNCH	DINNER	SNACK
MON				
TUE				
WED				
THU				
FRI				
SAT				
SUN				

IMPORTANT NOTES

SHOPPING LIST

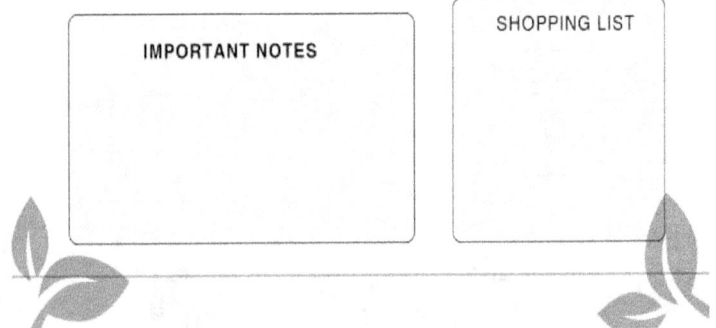

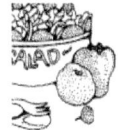 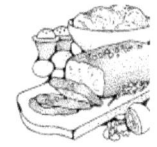

WEEKLY MEAL PLANNER

MONTH:

WEEK:

DAY	BREAKFAST	LUNCH	DINNER	SNACK
MON				
TUE				
WED				
THU				
FRI				
SAT				
SUN				

IMPORTANT NOTES

SHOPPING LIST

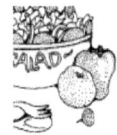 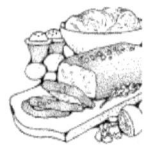

WEEKLY MEAL PLANNER

MONTH:

WEEK:

DAY	BREAKFAST	LUNCH	DINNER	SNACK
MON				
TUE				
WED				
THU				
FRI				
SAT				
SUN				

IMPORTANT NOTES

SHOPPING LIST

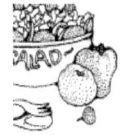 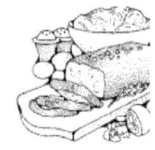

WEEKLY MEAL PLANNER

MONTH:

WEEK:

DAY	BREAKFAST	LUNCH	DINNER	SNACK
MON				
TUE				
WED				
THU				
FRI				
SAT				
SUN				

IMPORTANT NOTES

SHOPPING LIST

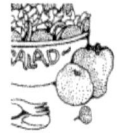 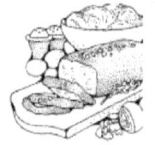

WEEKLY MEAL PLANNER

MONTH:

WEEK:

DAY	BREAKFAST	LUNCH	DINNER	SNACK
MON				
TUE				
WED				
THU				
FRI				
SAT				
SUN				

IMPORTANT NOTES	SHOPPING LIST

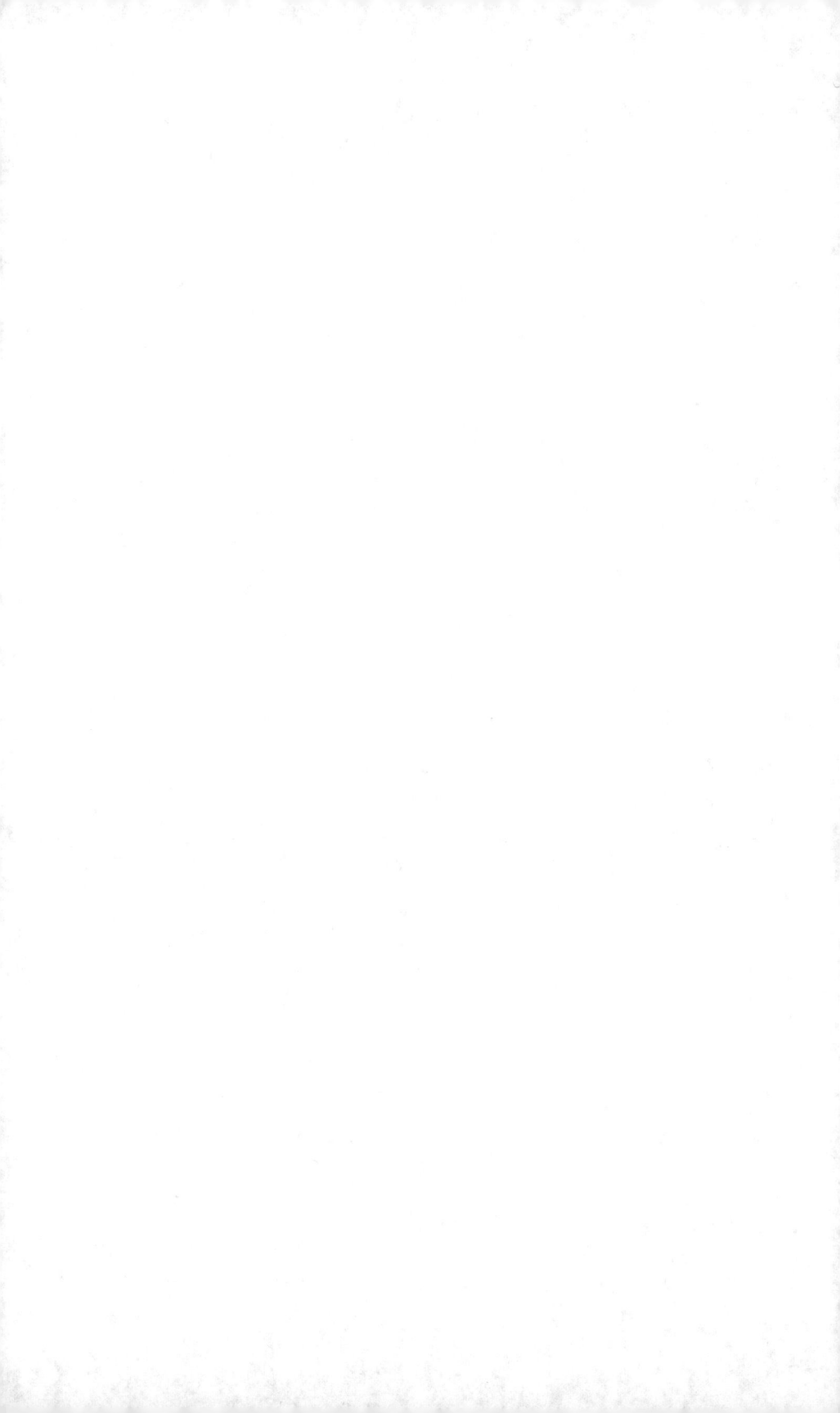

www.ingramcontent.com/pod-product-compliance
Lightning Source LLC
Chambersburg PA
CBHW062331290526
45794CB00005B/1983